LET ME DOWN
EASY

LET ME DOWN EASY

ANNA DEAVERE SMITH

THEATRE COMMUNICATIONS GROUP
NEW YORK
2018

The publication of *Let Me Down Easy* by Anna Deavere Smith, through TCG's Book Program, is made possible in part by the New York State Council on the Arts with the support of Governor Andrew Cuomo and the New York State Legislature.

TCG books are exclusively distributed to the book trade by Consortium Book Sales and Distribution.

Library of Congress Control Numbers:
2017056190 (print) / 2017061736 (ebook)
ISBN 978-1-55936-546-8 (trade paper) / ISBN 978-1-55936-867-4 (ebook)
A catalog record for this book is available from the Library of Congress.

Cover, book design and composition by Lisa Govan
Cover photo by Joan Marcus

First Edition, June 2018

This play is dedicated to the memories of
Governor Ann Richards, Reverend Peter Gomes, Joel Siegel,
Hazel Merritt and Anna Young Smith

Contents

LET ME DOWN
EASY

Let Me Down Easy was originally presented Off-Broadway at Second Stage Theatre (Carole Rothman, Artistic Director), opening on October 8, 2009. It was directed by Leonard Foglia; the set design was by Riccardo Hernandez, the costume design was by Ann Hould-Ward, the lighting design was by Jules Fisher and Peggy Eisenhauer, the original music was composed by Joshua Redman, the sound design was by Ryan Rummery; the dialect coach was Amy Stoller, the movement coach was Elizabeth Roxas-Dobrish, the dramaturg was Alisa Solomon, the projection designer was Zak Borovay, and the production stage manager was Kelly Martindale. The show was conceived, written, and performed by Anna Deavere Smith.

Note from the Playwright

To enhance the reader's frame of reference, sometimes physical descriptions are given—including age, body size, and race. These are not meant to suggest casting. I perform the play as a one-person show. Audiences may or may not have thought about these details while observing my performance. It is my intention that, eventually, casts of any size, age group, or ethnicity will be able to perform the play. The director may choose to cast people according to actual age, race, or physical type. That could, of course, make for an interesting production. However, there is also the option to cast roles against expected type. Details of physique, age, and race are provided to give information and clues about the person's worldview. These are real people who live or did live in the real world. I have also sometimes included the date of the interview, in order to suggest the cultural, political, and social environment in which the interview took place.

The notes are sometimes less actual stage directions and more an attempt to give the performers the "actual scene" of the originating interview. Therefore, there may be props or actions denoted that were in the real scene but not in Mr. Foglia's stage production. All utterances, including non-words such as "um"s and "uh"s should be spoken, as they create the scansion of the text. The text is as much an observation of identity through utterance as it is a descant on the human body, its vulnerability, and its resilience.

James H. Cone

Author, Reverend, and Professor
Union Theological Seminary, New York City

"Let Me Down Easy"

African-American man, seventy years old, great shape, a runner, in a
colorful shirt with no tie, jeans.

Let me down easy. You know that's, that's, those are words;
those are words [of a] broken heart. They *can* be interpreted
as broken love. And I certainly heard it within that context.

Let me down easy. That's about love broken. Don't do it so
harshly. Don't do it too mean. Let it be easy. And, but as most
people realize, most of that: black love songs and blues and jazz
is a transmutation of, about injustice too. But it's, but it's covert.
Not overt. And it's a combination of, of, of, of talking about
love. And at the same time talking about hurt *from* broken love.
Brokenheartedness. And at the same time, hurt from what's happening to you in society. So it's a. But it certainly is about love.
When I think about it. People-need-something-to-sustain-them-
in-times-of-difficulty.

Whether that's personal, whether that's social, they need that something *within* that you can't always explain. That something within you, that is a kind of affirmation *of* you. And it enables you to know who you are, and be at peace with who you are, at ease with who you are, no matter what's happening around you and no matter what you're going to face! You know, that keep on gittin' on!

Hmm, it could be related to *[death]* too. Could be about dying. "Let me die easy, when I die." Yeah, it could mean that. Yeah, it could mean that. That's the thing about language in the black community. It has many meanings and uh, yeah, it could, it could definitely mean that. "Swing low sweet chariot, coming for to carry me home"? Yeah, yeah, that's right. It could mean that.

Elizabeth Streb

Choreographer, STREB Dance Company, New York City

"Fire Dance"

At her action studio, white woman in her fifties, very physically fit, wearing an oversized, extravagant-looking man's suit, Mohawk hairstyle, lots of gel, heavy motorcycle boots, wearing a large peace sign and intense designer black-framed glasses.

About death? First thing I think about is I have *ways* I'd like to die? Like I'd like to—I mean one time I was on fire. Because I did a fire dance for my girlfriend? And I caught on fire accidentally. And I thought, "I don't think I would want to burn to death." I accidentally caught on fire. I used Sterno, I used Sterno, I'm crazy. This was a couple years ago.

This was a couple years ago and I wanted to make something for her fortieth birthday that was *really* special. For Laura, yeah. And so I thought of "Blaze Away"? Where basically I'd start a fire and then I'd fall on it and put it out? And so I used the Melissa Etheridge song? *(She sings one line)* *"'Cause I'm the only one who'd walk across the fire for you-hoo."*

So I made Laura stand at that end and I stood here. And my dancers were lighting the fire. And I made her walk *towards* me and.

She had no idea what I was doing. And there were like a hundred people at the party. And uh, I'd rehearsed it so . . . And I flew in, you fly, you go into a crouch. And at this certain moment you go into a fly . . . into a flying horizontal X? And land on . . . I made the fire as big as this torso part so I would *(Smacking her hands together loudly)* smoosh it—but big enough that you see the fire but not so big that it went outside my body— because I would just *smoosh* the oxygen out of it. And I landed on it. But unbeknownst to me—I'd been rehearsing? And had some Sterno on my torso? So when I went like, "Woom!" Like that—and I looked under and I go, "Oooh, uh—oh, I'm on fire." And, "Ooh," I smooshed it! And I go, "Oh! That's not gonna happen."

So I stood up and I was literally on fire. And I mean I was just like—then I went like this—and, *"Oh my god, that is the fastest phenomenon I've ever seen. I've never seen anything move that fast, be that fast."* And, you know, I was like, *"Okay."* And just the seconds were stretched? And like everyone, *everyone* in the room was look- ing at me: like, "Oh my god!" But nobody did *anything*. Because— Yeah! Isn't it fucking crazy? Did nothing, they just like, and even my friend was continuing to take *pitchers [sic]*, Danita, my friend! And I was like going, *"Okay."* And then I was sort of going like *this*. And I was saying, "Well that's not gonna work." This Sterno's gonna burn—because it went through my pants—this Sterno's gonna burn, until it's gone, right? But the thing is, it was travel- ing *up* my body? And if it got to my hair, I was thinking I would, the thing I was thinking was I'd ruin Laura's party? Because I'd be whisked away to the ambulance—

So my dancers, who do call-and-respond; we do call-and- respond. They know. They go, *"Take-it-OFF!"* And Terry Dean grabbed my ankles, my ankles of my pants, and I jumped up, and he took off the pants, and I ran out of the room, and it was over. I just had a little burn.

But it was really one of the most profound experiences 'cause, you know, I felt like, for a few days I'd see complete strangers and just, I'd think to myself, "Well, you know, I've been on fire. I was on fire." So. It's that kind of thing.

I would love to have—I'd like to know what it feels like to get shot. I would like a rough trauma kind of injury: fall—like falling a long ways and crashing. Like I think I'd like that. Or I'd like maybe to explode, do it quicker.

You know, there are just some people that really embrace the danger thing. They're not worried about hurting themselves. I think that people tend to worry about hurting themselves . . . and I think that, I think that's a class thing? Like how much, how many feet of protection does who get, on earth? How high are their fences? Like the people who are the richest are the furthest away from any type of penetration.

The poorest people, you know, have scars on their face? Because they, they can't keep harm away from them. And so the whole relationship to harm, and to what you're willing to take, that whole thing: "Oh death, where is *[thy]* sting-a-ling-a-ling?" How *alive* do you wanna be? I'd like to die in the middle of a move basically. That's how I'd like to die, in the middle of a move.

Well, what about you, how would you like to die? *(Pause, waiting)* Oh come on! Don't you want to know the lights are gonna go out in a particular way? Does it scare you, the idea of dying? *(Pause)* It's sad, right?

LANCE ARMSTRONG

Tour de France Victor

"Right on Time"

March 2007. A suite at the Pierre Hotel, New York City. He is barefoot, bright blue T-shirt, athletic shorts that come to his knee. A few seconds of music by Ben Harper playing. He turns off the music.

I did not spend a lot of time thinking about that. There, there were just the, well there would have been these moments where you thought, "Oh no, yeah, I'm gonna die." But they didn't last long. Well ya, ya had these peaks where: So you're diagnosed, "Oh shit. I'm gonna die." And, it's all over your lungs, "Oh no, now I'm *really* gonna die." And by the way, it's in the brain, "Yah, now I'm *really* gonna die." But those, those didn't last long. It was just like, almost like an EKG, you know, just like these little things were *(Demonstrates EKG data going up and down with his forefinger)* and then they quickly went away and I got back into the mode of, of being treated an', an', an' focusing on that.

So and then, that was supported by the blood work that would follow. So tumor markers *in* the blood, saying, you know, lower and lower and lower and lower. Doctor's happy, on course for a "cure." A chest X-ray you could actually look at, which is pretty cool. So you see a golf ball, that turns to a marble, that turns into a pebble, then goes away. I got it, I mean, I can see that! Um, so that encourage—that encouragement, that was, *that* was my inspiration, my motivation.

You mean the *[medical]* team *during* the disease? Well I didn't know anything about the disease, so I had no choice but to quickly figure out what a team was. And before that I had been a good athlete and part of a team sport, but I didn't really know the true definition of team. So we quickly put together a few key friends and family members that then finds very key and critical caregivers: doctors, nurses, researchers.

And this all the while when it was hard to find that stuff. This was ten years ago. It was not the internet age. But finally puttin' together a team that you could believe in, the ones 'at—with the highest—stakes—on the line—your life.

(Brief pause. Then in a monotone:)

It was a bit of a shock, taught me a lot. *[When I got back into cycling]*, just like you would with the disease, we looked at every little aspect. And I had not done that before in, in cycling. And then when I came back, uh, we looked at every aspect. So everybody involved, every individual involved was sort of handpicked or analyzed.

And then, uh, then I think that, ultimately, the, the, the overarching thing was just this fear of failure that I learned, or *had* to learn when I was sick because, you know, people say, "Why were you motivated to win? Was it fame? Was it money? Was it, uh, whatever—was it a *trophy*?" Uh, whereas with the disease, uh I mean, the fear there, the motivation is failure, 'cause failure's death. And so I took that into cycling. Not that I thought I was gonna *die* if I lost the Tour. But I certainly—I didn't—I just didn't want to face this, this, this *demon* called failure.

You mean like on a, on a spiritual level? *(Laughs)* I'm not very spiritual. In fact, I'm not spiritual at all. Other than to say,

I mean, I think that I have a right to be a good and decent and honest person and I mean it could be called, it could be called karma.

I cannot be the guy that just completely goes around and, I could never've been the person goes around and just screws people. I mean I feel like I have an obligation to do the right thing.

An obligation as an athlete, as a cancer survivor, as a father, as a friend . . . as a husband, as a boyfr—or whatever. And I've made mistakes, trust me.

Uhhhhhhh, but I mean I, I never looked at it uh, uh, uh, uh, again from a religious standpoint. Other than to say I have what I have . . . and I feel like I have a responsibility to, to, to be something. While I'm here. On this planet.

I felt a little, uh, responsible to be productive. I felt responsibility. For that. Sport, the disease, kids.

It's tough.

It's tough as I—

I think it's tough as life gets bigger and, and life becomes more complicated.

You know it's not easy to be present. I mean that's the mo— that's the best thing you can do for somebody is be present, I mean I'm sitting here, I could be sitting here reading my BlackBerry and and looking at the *New York Post* and you're like: "The fuck's this guy doing?" But, you know, you sit down, and—if you're going to be there you're there. If you're sitting with your kids, if you sit down to the, to the dinner table, which is one of the three most important things you can do with 'em, you're there. Dad is there. Ask about the spelling test, ask about . . . your girlfriend, ask about whatever, you're the—Dad's there. Dad's not . . . you know. Talking to the cook or the the nanny or the, looking outside at the sunset, Dad's there!

I've never felt bad about being ultra-competitive. I never felt like I was putting somebody out of work or out of their home.

I didn't care. Heh-heh. Quite honestly, I didn't care.

Maybe, uh, maybe 'cause the, the, the, the hyper-competitiveness came from the disease, just because there, the stakes were so high. I mean, somebody was trying, something or somebody was trying to put me out of work forever. So.

And if you win four or five or six of them, there's history on the line. And I was aware of that.

Look, there were people denied a lot of great opportunities. There was a guy who was five times second in the Tour de France. Sucks to be him.

But, I look at it as, uh, he didn't make the sacrifices that I made. He didn't do the things that I did, didn't have the work ethic that I had, didn't have the *team* that I had. So, that's what you get.

(Hotel doorbell rings.)

Your berries are coming. *(Teasing)* That's probably our breakfast. *(To the waiter)* Hi. *(He gets up and comes back with a tray of berries and muffins)* Eat your berries.

I thought we were on our last questions! *[Now wait a second]* I can't talk forever. I told you I hate interviews. Three more questions, please.

(Breaks a muffin in half with his hands, eats. Stands up, looks at a bank of microphones on the coffee table.)

Jesus! You think you got enough microphones? So what are you gonna do with all this?

(Listens and responds:)

What do you mean?
     I've never seen a play. What do you mean?
     So, you mean like a play in New York?
     Okay, for starters? I cannot sit through a movie. But I'll go.
     They don't last more than a couple of hours do they?
     You should interview my mom. She'll talk to you if I tell her to, yeah. She's, she's great; she's very, very uh, five-foot-three, hundred pounds. Ten-pound baby boy. Came the day he was due.
     Did you come the day you were due?
     You were early?
     I was right on time!

Sally Jenkins

Sports Columnist, Washington Post

"Ashes"

September 2007 and August 2009. Sitting in her apartment, overlooking the Hudson River, New York City, white woman in her forties, flip-flops, several stacked rings on left hand, plays with rings. Has a large mug of tea.

There is something in an athlete like that—who understands that they were perfectly built for this job, for this task. There is a feeling of completion that they're driven to.

I mean it's kind of like they are going to fulfill this destiny and fulfill this body—

It's, it's very hard to articulate, but I think that when you're given that body, or those skills, you've been given kind of this emotional component as well—try and stop 'em!

It's, it's, it's like nuclear fusion! It's *(Pausing in wonder)* like—it's like nuclear fusion! I think it might be a natural force. The laws of physics are gonna take over.

Lance *[Armstrong]* is all about releasing energy. He can't even, he could not even sit. in. this. chair. and have this conversa-

19

tion. He *drives* like a bat out of hell. Every athlete I've ever known drives a hundred miles an hour.

Pat Summitt *[University of Tennessee basketball coach]* drives to work from her house—she's not even an athlete anymore, she's a coach—she drives, she has got her foot down on the gas, and she's putting mascara on and she's driving—she's *steering* with her knee—and she's going like this, and she's putting on her makeup and getting ready to go coach a ball game, she's got four things on the stove—she's stirring them all—she probably scrubbed the baseboards before she left, because there's just this *force*.

Downhill skiers drive a hundred twenty miles an hour. They're all—that's why with this whole doping thing, it's ridiculous to say to them, "Oh, don't do that, you might *hurt* yourself!" *(Laughs heartily, loudly)*

Tell a downhill skier, tell an Austrian gold-medalist, downhill Olympic skier, "Oh no! You don't want to take a little EPO. You might *hurt* yourself!" Are you *kidding* me?

They don't understand it. It's patronizing. Some guy told me that the Greeks would have ground up rhinoceros skin and eaten it if they thought it would make them run any faster or do anything any better. It's like, I remember watching this documentary on the, Stephen Hawking's book? The—'member his, his, the, his book for—Hawking . . . What was the, what the hell is the name of that book? I'm not remembering. Was a good little documentary about it and there was a great little part of this documentary where they show what—the energy that's released when just a cup breaks . . . You drop, if I drop this cup to the floor and it breaks. And there was this great illustration of, of the energy that's released and how it—the, the cup—has to fall, and it has to *(Slapping her hands together with force)* hit the floor; and the energy is released and you can't get it back again. You can't, the teacup can't come back up from the floor and put itself back together again. That's not how matter works. Well, those are athletes! Athletes are the cup dropping to the floor and smashing.

I mean they are there to fulfill absolutely everything that's in them. So, you know, athletes—a lot of athletes—will tell you, "It's not the winning, it's the trying." And it's a cliché but happens to be very true. You know, athletes are about exhausting themselves. You know, they're not happy until they're absolutely used up. And people get real uncomfortable with that because they want to see them and remember them at their peak? Athletes themselves want to turn to *ashes*. To an athlete, there's nothing worse than cheating their body; they're cheating their, uh, destiny or cheat . . . You know, that—that failure to use everything they have, is, is the ultimate sin to somebody like Lance Armstrong. It's why they come back. They can't walk away feeling like there's anything left in the tank. And that's Lance—to walk around feeling like there's a third of a tank? Can't, can't live that way.

Mean to me, an athlete has two deaths. Bill Bradley said that one time, you know. When an athlete retires—when they, when they, when someone like Lance reaches the end of his road; it's a form of death. Certainly is a, a form of surrender. That's why they have such a hard time with it. And they don't want that incarnation of themselves to die.

We don't want that incarnation of them to die.

People want perfection from athletes, and they want moral perfection from athletes. As spectators we want to, we want to keep this vision of them as sort of perfect for all time; we want them to be immortal, you know, in our eyes.

And so then when someone like Lance comes along, lot of people go well ah—you know, "I don't want to remember him as less than great," you know, or, "Why is he tainting his legacy?" . . . all that nonsense you know. But I think it's because people, I think people want perf—you know, that kind of timeless perfection. And, it makes them uncomfortable, to watch athletes grow old. I mean, athletes are *us*.

EVE ENSLER

Writer, Activist

"A Raisin a Day"

December 2007. On a sofa, in the living room of her apartment in New York City, small cup of espresso, stack of rings on right hand.

Why don't we want to see women age? Why, why is everyone so terrified to see women age?

Why are we so terrified to see aging period in this culture?

Why do we put old people in places and remove them from sight? Because they remind us: "I'm gonna die." They remind us that: "We're leaving here." And I think that's true with the body!

If you have the perfect body and perfect *tits* and perfect *ass*, it moves you forward with *men*. It moves you forward with *women*. It moves you forward in *jobs*. And I think fitting yourself into that idea has become what people are spending a lot of time doing. You know, just money, energy, attention, time. *(Smacking hands together)*

But it's also connected to dying. Very much connected to dying.

Because I think in this culture people don't really die. See, death isn't amongst us. Death isn't with us. We're all immortal here. We are all forever young here. We're all, and I think so—if you can control your body and manipulate your body and designate your body, and it's all part of this whole immortal . . .

Like the reason I believe in sex. Like, above everything in the whole world, like the reason I think sex is so important—is that—it's where you see your body—in relationship to another body. But where you can . . . ah! It's just genius, sex, because it's where it becomes spiritual—and it's where it becomes intellectual—and where the body starts morphing into all these other amazing things. And I think—often girls get cut off from sexuality at a very young age. And so that is what then directs them to start manipulating their bodies.

It's almost like anorexia is a kind of a very asexual thing. Those aren't the girls having sex. Those are the girls fixing their body. There's sex. And there's *fixing* your body. I am making a piece about teenage girls. I am obsessed with teenage girls.

It's really about coming into your power. Coming into your voice. Coming into your sexuality, coming into your wet, fluid, gushy life, and going, "Oh my . . . god. I got to get rid of it." Because it's such a threat to the culture. It's such a threat to everything. And so what you learn how to do, because capitalism teaches you this, because the commodified culture is structured on this . . . is getting rid of the *mess* where the *mess* would actually *allow* you to be a human, which would allow you to protest, which would allow you to revolt, which would allow you to have passion, which would get you to go out and somehow reconstruct the system. But if you keep shutting the person down, and limiting the person, then you disappear the person.

You get to be that skinny, you get to be that disappeared— All these girls who are starving themselves—I mean, you can't *think* much when you've eaten a raisin a day. You know, you're not producing a lot of *thought*. You know, you need *food* in order to have a thought. So it's like, you just keep shutting the system out, shutting the system out and shutting the sys—so that you're finally not a threat to anybody. So that you're disappeared.

And I don't—think—that's—accidental—one—tiny—bit.

I think it comes from capitalism! I think capitalism's actually, the motor of this system is: "How do you keep people hooked on a disappearing idea of themselfs *[sic]*?"

The people I *most* am drawn to are the women who actually— I used to have like this little game I play, like, "Who Lives in Their Vagina." And I would watch people walking down the street. And watch people and I *[would]* go: "In her vagina. Not in her vagina. In her vagina . . ."

Like Tina Turner? *In!* Implanted! Illuminated! Transcendent! You know, and you can watch her career where she literally *lands* in her vagina. Like you know, you know, she was in her vagina when she was younger. But then she really *landed* in her vagina when she got to be in her fifties. When "What's Love Got to Do with It," after she left Ike? There was just like, oh my *god*! And I used to go and sit in the *third* row of all of her concerts, just so it would be kind of, I would osmos *[sic]* her, living in her vagina into me.

That's what it looks like! That's what it feels like! If you're actually, fully, incarnated in your body!

BRENT WILLIAMS

Rodeo Bull Rider, Idaho

"Toughness"

August 2003 and September 2009. At a nearly empty rodeo ring in Sho-shone, Idaho, midday. A stunningly attractive, rugged white male in his twenties in a cowboy hat, boots, jeans, long-sleeved shirt. There are bulls grazing in a closed area. People on horses, practicing. Drinking a Bud Light.

I got hung up by a bull, weighed over a ton. *[Bull stepped on my back, in the rodeo.]* It wasn't a mean bull, but when I hit the ground, I was on my side and he stepped on my left side with two back feet, broke, uh, four ribs, L2, L3, and there was a guy, the urologist for the hospital was sitting in the front row when I got stepped on. And he came back and he told me, "Kid, you better go to the hospital." He said, "I bet your kidney or your spleen's ruptured." I was like, "Ah no, I just broke some ribs."

Said, "No, I'm serious, you need to get this checked out. I'm serious. I'm a urologist *[at]* a military hospital."

He got on the phone and called the hospital. A civilian can only go to a military hospital if it's a life-or-death situation and he called and told them, you know, that it is a life-or-death situation.

I was kind of laughing. I didn't believe him, you know. They took me to the hospital and had me piss in a cup and it was just straight red blood. Brooke Army Medical Center in San Antonio, Texas.

Whole time I'm just thinking, "How long I have to sit out before I can rodeo again?" About an hour later they told me that they were gonna have to remove my left kidney.

I begged them for an hour. Said, "I wanna ride bulls and if I only had one kidney—I'd just as soon have two." They tried a new deal. They put a stent in there. That saved half my kidney, so I got one-and-a-half kidneys, instead of one.

[And] them guys get paid a flat rate, it's not like they're tryin' to rape me to make more money to pay their Mercedes-Benz bills or whatever they got. And I'll bet you most of those guys don't even drive them fancy sports cars like the doctors do. Cost me a flat rate: twelve hundred bucks.

Yah, twelve hundred bucks, flat rate. Didn't matter if I got CAT-scans or whatever they did to me. And I didn't, it didn't change when I was in ICU for six days, and then when they took me to the next level. It didn't change. I didn't get no doctor bills or nothing. And I was in there for eleven days. Everyone, everyone pays a flat rate, no matter what it is. I, I *[personally]* think we need to go to a deal like *[that]*.

And I think, and I think I had better doctors there that wanted to be doctors instead of these pricks these days that just go to college and spend all their parents' money going to college and then they make a killing and they don't really give a shit. You tell me a poor doctor and I'll kiss his ass. We'll see what doctors really wanna be doctors when there's not as much money in it.

And them doctors, I felt like, well they told me if I'd a went to the other hospital in San Antone *[sic]*, if it had been anywhere else, they'd a just took my kidney out. So I'm very grateful for them doctors.

(Pause, listening.)

Yeah, I've got insurance. I have a family policy for, through Blue Cross of Idaho. Two hundred, two hundred sixty bucks a month, to cover all of us and it's like seventy-five-hundred-dollar deductible. Which is stupid. We don't ever meet that, I mean all this paying money and then, you know, 'cause we got to pay seventy-five hundred before they meet it.

I mean, all they do is they rape us. They, it's just like all the people that got the money. They rape the poor, until they, or they rape the middle class, until the middle class becomes poor. Then they'll start raping the rich. I mean they're gonna, they're gonna break the whole country I think.

But basically I'm an optimist.

(Pause.)

You know when, when you ride a bull and you do good and ride them . . . You feel like, you know, like there ain't nothing in this world that could probably you know, you know, beat you up. Or anything like that, you know, you just feel like life couldn't be better, you know, like this is, that's what life's supposed to be. Feels, I don't know, 'cause there's like so much power. You know, if you think about it, you shouldn't be able to stay on the back of a bull that's trying to buck you off! You know, 'cause we weigh a hundred and fifty pounds, you know, and they weigh two thousand pounds, you know.

You feel like a king at the moment you know. Yeah, you know.

(Pause.)

You can't stay on top of *every* bull. I think it comes from inside you, what keeps you on that bull, you know, I think it's determination.

I mean Pat O'Mealy, my wife's uncle, gave me my first cotton flanker rope. He always said, "Kid, you got more try than anybody I have ever seen." And try and determination is the same thing.

When I'm not rodeoin' no more? I'll be all right, I have my ranch and my cows and all that. I don't want to think about when that day comes. There'll just be like an empty, a big ol' empty space in me, I think. Probably like maybe an even bigger empty space in me than when like my brother died.

You know, I don't know for sure, you know, how it'll be, you know. That was a pretty big empty space. But I guess I feel like when I'm done rodeoin', it probably be like the day my brother died, you know.

Toughness?

We's in West Jordan, Utah. And I had this bull shove my face like right through the metal chutes. I mean my nose . . . took like five hours to sew me up. My buddies took me to the hospital. When they straightened my nose, I *[had to]* be at a rodeo that night I didn't really want to go under the an-es-theez-ya, or however you say that word. So I told them just to do it without it.

They shove these two rods up your nose and work their way up and that straightens your nose all up. Felt like they was shoving it clear through my brains an' it was gonna come out the top of my head. And everyone that saw it, they said it should have killed me. And they didn't even knock me out. So I guess that'd be toughness.

But once they did that, I could breathe. And I hadn't been able to breathe *[through my nose]* since I had broke it when I was, like, in high school rodeo!

MICHAEL BENTT

World Champion Heavyweight Boxer

"When Boxers See Lights"

Former heavyweight champion. Charismatic African-American man. On a boxing stool, with a bottle of water. Wearing a hooded sweatshirt, hood down on shoulders, chewing gum. Boxing gear in a large athletic bag nearby: mitts, cell phone, a small towel. A jump rope beside the bag. He speaks very softly, except where otherwise noted. Actor should strive for every word, especially the "You know"s, "Like, you know"s, etc.

When I fought Tommy Morrison, he was like, he was like our version, this generation's version of *The Great White Hope*. He beat George Foreman in twelve rounds in 1993. And I was Tommy's quote-unquote tune-up match to his fight. Prior to fighting Lennox Lewis for eight-point-five-million dollars. Tommy was sharp, good-looking cat. Put asses in seats.

(Phone rings, he checks it, ignores it.)

And I was just a good amateur. Had a soft chin. Call it weak whiskers. HBO had a free date and they wanted to fill it just to keep

Tommy sharp. When I signed the fight I'm like, first of all, "Ain't no white boy beating me. Not in Tulsa." *(Phone rings)* It's the wife. *(Smiles)* Hey Lees, hey baby. I'm with Anna okay? Can I talk to you in a little bit? Okay, baby. *(Turns off phone)*

Well, I mean, the way I understand athletics to be, you have to damn near kill a white boy to get a decision. Absolutely, absolutely. I mean, the judges and referees are white. But I'm not saying the majority of fans don't appreciate a Muhammad Ali or a Ray Robinson. But I think when those fighters fight a white fighter they abandon their admiration.

Well, for me, and uh, that night, that shit motivated me. I mean, I'm in this boy's backyard? Tulsa, Oklahoma? And I'm fighting a white boy? Whoo! Naw-unh! And my thinking was, "Not on my watch."

(Takes towel out of bag, hangs it, folded vertically, in waistband of pants.)

I was ready to die. Sure! Yeah! That night. He was gonna have to kill me.

(Responding to a question) Oh yeah, absolutely, yeah, yeah. And you know what, Anna, honestly? When I got hit by Tommy in the first round? When I hit the rope I was going down. I mean, the rope saved me. *(Puts on mitts)* If the rope wasn't there—I got knocked down. I was *out*. The first thought when I hit that rope: "You cannot go back to Queens having a white boy beat you." It was like those, those, those, those, uh those signs, uh, um, that uh, you know that, post the uh, the uh *Wall Street* listings? You know I mean? You cannot go back to Queens with a white boy beating you.

In preparation for the fight, uh, I watched Tommy's fights like you know, *maniacally*. And I would realize when he got somebody hurt, he would stop breathing.

He would, he would panic essentially. And he would: *(Sucks in air and holds breath)*

And, ah throw punches, like wow! "This fool, like, you know, doesn't know how to finish somebody." He gets excited, like when, like you know, he has a guy hurt. Doesn't know how to finish. So I get hurt. Uh, thirty seconds into the fight. And I'm um, I'm hurt bad. It's a temple shot. But he, I, me, he knows I'm hurt and he tries, he tries to finish me. And stops breathing. So he's tight. In his, uh, enthusiasm to like, you know, finish me for his hometown crowd? I threw a right hand and connected right on the point of the chin. Which is like, you know *(Sucks air in)* the bull's-eye *(Sucks air in)* in boxing, you know. Um, and he, he drops. Gets back up. Um, I drop him again and he got back up again. And I dropped him again. And it was, you know, they stop the fight after three knockdowns. And I won like, you know, uh-uh-um-uh, a piece of the World Heavyweight Championship.

I took out my mouthpiece, and I threw it. And I started crying, I started crying. Bawled like a child. I don't know if it was the pressure of beating a white boy. Or the pressure from my father—

My father, man, I mean, was a very, very proud Jamaican man. *(Mimicking a Jamaican accent, very loudly)* "This is my son Mikahl Bentt, thuh Boxah!" When I was growing up, I used to resent that shit, because, he would come home after hanging with his friends and make me jump rope for them. Skip rope for them. He was just proud that his son could skip rope like Muhammad Ali, but, when you're ten years old, you don't want to be awakened at four o'clock in the morning, made to skip rope for strangers. Can you imagine? "MIKE!" It would terrify me, man, because I'd be in a deep sleep. *(Jamaican accent, very deep register)* "MIKE! MICHAEL! WAKE UP AND BRING YOUR ROPE, YOUR JUMP ROPE." "Okay, Daddy, I'm coming, I'm coming." And sometimes, I fall back asleep. "MIIIIIKE!" You know, when my father would get loud, the whole house would shake. It was like Othello loud. Like you knew it was going to be chaos, somebody was going to get fucked up, somebody was going to feel some pain.

So, I win a World Championship, and ten minutes later I'm like sitting in the locker-room and everybody's like, you know, there's like, you know, minor pandemonium, you know what I mean? You know, minor, like, you know, everybody was like, "Hey, Mike, how ya doin'?" I'm like, This is such bullshit. Such bullshit. *(Beat)* Fuck am I doing here?

Yeah, I box because my dad wanted me to be a boxer, you know what I mean? And I wanted to be a blay—a baseball player. *(Pause)*

You know. Or a fuckin' writer. I don't know. You know maybe like, you know, I could been, like, you know, a great piano player, uh, like you know a great pianist, who—who knows? But like, you know, I didn't want to box. Who wants to get, um, like, who wants to get hit?

But my last fight? *[I don't remember it at all.]* The Herbie Hide thing!

Last thing I remember was being in a, uh, in a hotel? You familiar with London at all? In the Isle of Dogs, um, an' um. I'm eatin' pasta and there was like a, a, a, a, a, a, a um, a platoon of FOI. The English, um, um, members of the Nation of Islam. *[I was a member of the Nation at the time.]* You know, my, my, my, my, entourage, as it were, you know.

[You] win a championship, buy a new *car.* You, you dumped *[sic]* your girlfriend for like, you know, a hot light-skinned sister. *(Laughs)*

No! I'm just kidding. No! *(Covers face with mitts)* I did, actually! *(Laughs very hard)* So I'm sitting there with my entourage, and I'm just eating pasta, and uh, trying to relax. And the next thing I remember is uh, uh, uh, um, I see like a little, a light. I'm like damn, "Am I knocked down?" I figure like, you know, that, that, that, that, that when boxers see lights, we figure like, "Well shit! I been knocked down." Right? 'Cause lights are typically on the ceiling, yeah? If I'm lookin' up, I must be on my back, right? So I'm looking at lights. Man! Uh sh—fuck! I try to get up. Shoulders, like you know, hands, you know, shove me back down. Or, or ease me back down. I see like, uh, the light, gets dimmer. And, instead of a series of lights it's one light. Am I bugging the fuck out? Am I high? What? Turns out it was a doctor's penlight. Um, my neurosurgeon was shining a penlight. And he said, uh, uh, uh, I think he said something like, "Mike, how are you? Do you know where you are?" I'm like, "Yeah I'm, I'm in London." Uh, uh, uh. And I think like, *[he said]* "'Member what happened to you?" "No, man." He said, "You got knocked out, was pretty bad. Herbie Hide. Seven rounds." I think I started crying.

I was, um, apparently—in um, I was um, uh, apparently in the hospital bed for like ninety-six hours. So like four days. In a coma. He said, "*[You]* got some swelling." Uh, um. "We were preparing you for, um, brain surgery, uh. But uh, the swelling went down." Uh, "And you," he said, uh, uh, "you can't fight anymore."

(He chews and stares at a point on the horizon, for thirteen seconds.)

You know, although I was conflicted about fighting, it defined me. You know, that was my, that was my, that was how I define myself, you know?

I walk into a room when I was champ, like, you know, people like, like was like, "Woo! That's Michael Bentt! World Heavyweight Champion, knocked out Tommy Morrison first round! Mike!" *(The word "Mike!" is very loud)*

You know, and people, you know bow down to *[you]*. Women now, they, they wou—would like, you know, would fawn. You know, um.

Couldn't fight anymore.

(Long pause.)

All right, that's cool.

HAZEL MERRITT

Patient, Yale–New Haven Hospital
(1945–2013)

"A Sheet Around My Daughter"

A heavy-set African-American woman in her late fifties. Bleached blond hair. Gray eyes. Earrings. Sparkly gold purse. In an immaculate, modern conference room at Yale–New Haven Hospital—referring to a video and still cameras that are recording her. Camera flashes.

Oh gosh. I, I would have went to the hairdresser's. *[I look] terrible!* I don't want to be on *camera*. Oh. Okay. So all I have to basically do is just answer your questions, is that it? So you can use our names in it? If you want, yeah, you could use, yeah, that would be all right. Yeah, yeah. *(Chuckling)* You could use my name, yes. Not my picture though. *(Laughs, wheezes)* I said not my picture though. *(Laughs)* 'Cause I look *terrible* today. I mean, it's all rainy and I just got up. Took a shower and ran, I just *ran* in here. Well, I didn't *run* but, I walked but. *(Slurps water. Clears throat and coughs with fist over mouth)* Hazel Merritt. H-A-Z-E-L Merritt. M-E-R-R-I-T-T. Licensed Ordained Evangelist.

37

Well I had pretty good health. Until 1989, when I was diagnosed with diabetes.

Now they're talking about my kidneys, and the word "kidney" was a very bad thing to hear. When he said that, "Your kidneys are," um, "are pretty bad and," uh, "eventually," um, "not right now, but somewhere along the road," he said, "in maybe one to two, maybe one to two years, or a year," or whatever he says. "I can't exact, exactly say when; you will go on dialysis. You will need dialysis," he says, "because kidneys, you know, they're just not gonna repair theirself," um, "and you will have to go on dialysis."

Well, that was very, very devastating. Uh, so, I says, "Dialysis! I'm not having any dialysis! I'm not having dialysis, Dr. Rastegar!"

And he says, "Well, let's-don't-you-know-just-talk-about-it-right-now-to-that-extent. Let's just see how everything goes, but *eventually*, you will, will have to have it." That was very very devastating, that I had actually reached a point where I had to have dialysis.

I respected Dr. Rastegar. I did. He's a very good doctor, more or less, in the sense that he listens, he does, but I really felt like I had to grab on to a higher power. I just had to grab a hold to faith.

At the time I had a *lot* to say. Yeah, I was telling him, you know, about my, um, about how my husband had died an' I told him about my daughter that had passed away.

(Pause, listening.)

My daughter had a different problem.

My daughter was smart, she was a very smart girl.

My daughter was twenty-four years old.

Matter of fact, she wanted to be a brain surgeon. She had more or less um, got out in the world and met the wrong kids . . . and she got tied up with some, the bad group and she got sick.

But she dated a fella, that *(Swallows)* was evidently infected, and she didn't know it, you know, and she—got the virus! It wasn't uh, intravenously, it was sexually. She had gotten very sick . . . And so I had some very bad experiences when my daughter went for her dialysis, when— But it didn't happen here at Yale, but it did happen at another hospital in New Haven, where my daughter went for her dialysis.

They hooked her up to the machine, and the nurses went down the other end of the hallway, and left her in a room on this machine and I sat there with her. And something happen. The thing came a loose and the blood went all over the whole room, all in my daughter's *hair*, all over her face, and I went running down the hall trying to find a nurse and I couldn't find the nurse. I looked in rooms. I was calling for help. And nobody came. For at least like about maybe I'd say every bit of about three to five minutes or five minutes it was a long *time*. And the blood was just coming out and coming out from the thing, and my daughter was just *crying* and the blood was all in her *hair*, all in her *face*, all on her *jeans*! And, um, you know, all *over*. It had gotten on me, it was squirting all over and it was like a *nightmare*.

So, finally when they come in they, um, wrap a sheet around her, on top of all the blood and unhook her from the, uh, machines and everything. And then tell me, well, I can "bring her back another day." And, uh, that, you know, she's soaking wet wit' blood and I can "bring her back another day." And, uh, you know, they'll "do the dialysis or whatever they were going to do another day." And I said, "Ohh—kay." And they just *put a sheet around my daughter. A sheet around my daughter.* And at the time I didn't have a car. Well, I had a car but it was in the shop. And we had to wrap her up in a sheet and with all the blood going through the sheet, and what not, and put her in a taxi, and bring her home. And so that made *[me]* have like a real bad, bad feeling about nurses and doctors. And how could they just do this?

I'm not saying it 'cause it was my daughter, but she was a very beautiful girl. And, uh, she died.

So I'm not having any dialysis.

LAUREN HUTTON

Supermodel

"Mojo"

The first "supermodel" in history. Dressed in a T-shirt and fatigue-like pants, bare feet, sitting on the floor in front of her sofa, New York City loft. A full tea set, pouring tea, rolling a cigarette out of cigarette papers and tobacco. Smokes in the course of it. Never stops moving throughout the monologue—always engaged in one of those two activities. Very energetic. Southern accent, deep voice. Speaks very fast. When modeling, Hutton was known for a broad smile.

If that happened to me? *Now? (Big sigh)* When I signed with Revlon, when I signed the first contract in modeling history, got a million dollars, that was nothing compared to what I really got. I had the flu! And Revson got all excited 'cause he was just signing away a million of his bucks, and he said, "Send her right now to the doctor!" And that's what I got paid in. I got *[paid in]* the best doctors in New York City. That's, I've always felt that that's what I really made from Revlon. I got connected. He sent,

Revson sent me to these guys and they sent me to each other. But I didn't even know them before I met Revson. Before I signed that contract I didn't know these doctors!

(Looking out at author's camera, which audibly clicks) Didn't, didn't, didn't, didn't, didn't flash. We notice all that. All the time. The best always knows the best! The best models know who the other best models are. We know. Because we've gone through the thinking of it, the science of it, the seeing of it, an' then, *[some of them]* are just genetic freaks who happen to be six-foot-four, or two, or whatever, an', one side of their face is the, looks like the other side, an', you know, they're just these exquisite, extraordinary E.T.s! So, they're accidents! But then there're other people who've *worked* it. And I'm sure the best violinists all know each other, the best doctors all know each other. And they, they pass you around! And I'm sure the best lawyers. Whoever, is, is, the profession, they all know each other.

And, you know, we're now, what? Seven billion people on the planet growing a million and a half a week? There are too many of us! There are too many of us! We are going to be in each other's *armpits* in seconds!

Anybody that can cut, or edge off any kind of value for themselves, be it money, be it fame, be it anything, gets a little edge into the best of whatever it is! Best ice cream, best bananas, best, *(Laughs)* you know, I mean, that's how we work! We have to sort of specialize.

(Pause as she finishes rolling cigarette, listens.)

Well, my value to me is, these are the only eyes I've got, this is all I see out of, is this shell here. I don't know. I don't know. I'm not who they think I am. *(Upbeat)* And I just thank God I, I know I'm with world-class doctors. I'm a stereotypical ignorant patient. I was from a working-class family, *serious*, working-class family. I just got lucky in that I changed classes. I don't ask them many questions. I ask what I can. But it just seems like, you know, you're asking them about, er, plant life on Mars! I don't know about plant life on Mars! I don't know what kind of oxygen they eat! I don't know anything so I don't know how to form a question. I know about weevils and rattlesnakes—

It's a, it's a, it's a suspicious thing *[medicine]*. It's a, it's, like, black magic. It's a, it's mojo. It's mojo. And it scares me and I don't scare easy. I really don't. Part of, was handed down from my mother! I remember her just thinking that a doctor was practically not human! They were in some sort of, you know, Super *Daddy* role! They were gods and Super *Daddy*. *(Laughing and showing that unforgettable smile)* And I remember hearing her voice change, when she'd be around doctors. And we had no money, but, that was one thing she did spend money on, was the occasional doctor. Well, I don't think they were very good doctors, but, the part of Tampa we lived in wasn't even incorporated yet, but we did get some doctors.

She *revered* the profession. It was like, it was like, you know, "Hubda, hubda, hubda," with some beads! It was a religious, you know, mania. It was religion! Absolutely. And then I would get to my own good doctors, I have zillions of questions, and I'd forget all the questions! And I'd get home and my friends would say, "Did you say this, did you, what, what about that?" And I would suddenly think, "Ooo! I forgot to ask them!" I don't have any language for it, but many times I've realized that when you go in to talk to a doctor, why waste your and *his* precious time? Write down the questions, and go in, and call them out! And say them out in whatever language you got! *(Slight pause)* And, I've almost never done that.

Certainly the part of the practice *[is]* the most money. Now, maybe a lot of my own good doctors, I didn't, certainly didn't have the most money of the people. I didn't even *know* these doctors before I signed that contract. Because Revson used to give millions and millions of dollars. Revson gave millions of dollars, back when millions were millions. *(Laughs)* Not the little lower-middle-class shit now. It was like serious money! You know, he'd give like ten million, twenty million bucks to medical institutions that were doing test work. Because I think most very rich guys want to live forever. And they give money to that purpose. That's, a very big goal. Live forever. And I, you know, so.

Ruth Katz

Patient, Yale–New Haven Hospital

"That Bedrock of Care"

Addressing the audience. White woman in her forties, red blazer-style jacket, jeans. Strong Jersey/Atlantic City accent.

I'm in a pretty unique position. But, despite that unique position, I certainly felt that I had to look out for myself and um, uh, make sure that things were done in a way I thought they should be done. That bedrock of care was there for me. Um, I don't think it's there for every patient—I'm—as we talked about. I had a, um, surgeon and an oncologist and a group of nurses in the oncology clinic, uh, and technicians, down in the, um, radiation therapy unit, and a, um, um, uh therapeutic radiologist. All of whom, um, uh gave me as much time as I needed to go through whatever questions I had, um, to, uh, and, to otherwise be supportive in whatever way, um, I felt I needed at the time.

Um, I got to spend a lot of time with these people. They gave me home numbers which I would never have abused and didn't.

Um, only called Barbara when I was running a certain fever that she wanted to know about. And whenever I talked to them, I felt like no question was stupid.

I've come to learn enough about the health-care system that, um, while I think doctors and nurses and institutions, even as wonderful as Yale is, um, make mistakes? Um, have their attention diverted, um, to other important tasks? Um and um, can't be there in, in every sort of way that you want them to be there.

As much faith as I have in this place, every time I got, um, chemotherapy and they give—I had a friend there with me. To make sure that the bag of chemotherapy with that *stuff* in there that *they're about to pump into me* was *exactly* what I was supposed to get. No more, and the right stuff!

I will tell you that when I, um uh, on the last drug, well, throughout the protocol, if your temperature went below, uh, went *above*, a hundred point two, no, I'm sorry, a hundred and *one* point two, um they wanted you to call. And, if it went high enough, they wanted you to come to the hospital and make sure nothing was wrong. Mine, at one point, had gone up to, um, close to a hundred and two. So I came in—and they admit you immediately to the oncology unit.

Um, and a, an oncology fellow, which is not a member of our full-time faculty, but someone who's in training here, specializing in oncology, came into my room:

"I want to apologize," um, "but we can't find your records. Could you tell me what kind of cancer you have?"

I said, "This is appalling." And he said: "Oh tha—hey, don'—it's not just *you*. That happens here quite a bit!" I said, "I'm appalled for *every patient who comes on this unit.*" And I had to go through from the beginning, my whole story!

Um, eventually, I will tell you as an aside. Um, eventually, I knew, I could tell by his questions, he was gonna get to the question of "Do-you-work?" And I have never advertised my position here, I just want to be treated like everybody else, um. And he said, "Do you work?" You know, about midway through these questions, and I said, "I do." He said, "Are you working full-time?" I said, "I am." He said, "*Where* are you working?" I said, "I'm associate dean at the medical school." And he said—now he looks up—an' he said, "At this medical school?" I said, "At the Yale School of Medicine." Um, he found my files within a half an hour.

KIERSTA KURTZ-BURKE

Physician, Charity Hospital, New Orleans

"Heavy Sense of Resignation"

Fall 2005. White woman in her thirties, sandals, simple clothes, in a disheveled ballroom in a fine hotel in New Orleans, in the French Quarter, after Hurricane Katrina.

You have people that start out assholes and they end up assholes. And they might even wind up bigger assholes because . . . The biggest asshole I met in my training experience? God! There's so many. Um. Mmm. God, it's so tough. Oh! I know. I remember him. Um, shit! I can't remember his name, but he was such an asshole.

He was a resident when I was a medical student. He was in OB/GYN, I think a lot of that OB/GYN stuff really like, kind of, hit a nerve with me. And he was fully planning, he was one of these guys who was like, "I can't wait to get out of Charity Hospital, this frickin' hellhole, these people—blah, blah, blah."

Probably the least pleasant part a my job *[at Charity Hospital, a public hospital in New Orleans]* —I see people who come in,

49

to train at Charity, like I always thought we had a tremendous opportunity to see what it would be like in some sense, without living it, to be poor—and to open up our *hearts* and our *minds* to these *fantastic* people coming into the hospital. Privileged students from all over, um, an' they come in to train, at Charity Hospital. They come in with their own baggage about what Charity Hospital is, or what, the Charity "population" is. You know, "our population." That's kind of a common phrase. It's like, "our population," meaning the people that we take care of and our distancing ourselves from them.

'Cause, you know, people come in with their own racism and their own classism and then . . .

This guy was fully intending to, you know, set up, I am sure, a very fancy, you know, he was constantly talking about, "Well, when I get out I'm not gonna have these kind of patients." You know, translation: poor, black, you know, no prenatal care—blah, blah, blah. One night we were on call—a young woman came in with pelvic inflammatory disease. So we were called to the emergency room. And it's tremendously painful to be examined when you have fulminant pel—pelvic inflammatory disease. And she was thirteen. She was there with an aunt. But her aunt was not in the room. In fact, I think—I think if I remember right this guy made her aunt *leave* the room. And he did a pelvic exam on her and she was so, in so much pain, and crying out. And he said to her, I want to get it right. *(Slight pause)* He said, "What's your problem?" *(Pause)* "Don't tell me that you haven't had something *bigger* than these two fingers up there, if you got this to begin with." *(Pause)* I mean he was my, uh, resident. So, you know, here I was, I was a medical student. I was a third-year medical student and he was a second-year resident, so he was many levels above me. I was so *shocked* and *crestfallen* and I was really.

Beat my myself up afterwards that I didn't, I don't know what. Punch him. You know, whatever. I did say to him after we were out of her, out of her earshot, "I cannot believe that you would treat someone like that. And I cannot believe—that is *disgusting* to me." And he said, and I remember this, he said to me, which is kind of the typical line, "Oh, you wait and see when

you're in my spot." You know this kind of *faux jaded* . . . thing.
Which is just, once you've been through this so many times, and
you've seen so many twelve year olds with pelvic inflammatory
disease, what? You become an asshole?

And I have to say, that one thing that I really loved about
being at Charity, is that I always thought, in my mind—so many
of the people that come through these doors, they have been
given the shit end of the stick in life, period. But you know what?
In my interaction with them, I can treat them like they are the
Saudi Arabian princess coming to Mayo Clinic. There's no reason that I can't provide the absolute, top-of-line, best medical
care for them.

And I think that was a very difficult thing, when things dete-
riorated in the hospital during Hurricane Katrina.

And that kind of veneer that you can take care of poor people, and you can take care of them as well as you can take care of
rich people—that veneer for me just fell.

One of my patients said to me, and he had lost, he had
already heard through family members that he had lost his
grandmother and his aunt. He's from the Ninth Ward, family
had gotten out, but *[he]* had lost his grandmother and his aunt.
I mean the water came up ten feet an hour in their house. And he
was really just grieving. Pretty young guy, like in his forties. And
he had a spinal cord injury and so he was pretty immobile, like
almost all my patients, very immobile. And he was just laying in
bed an' I just went in and we were talking and just sitting by his
bedside, an' you know, it's a hundred and six degrees, there are no
lights, we're reduced to feeding people very small portions, and
you know, I think I tried to keep a lot of, you know, stiff upper
lip in the first couple days, and cheery outlook with the patients.
"Hey, you know, we're going to get out of here, don't worry about
it—blah, blah, blah."

And I think we were all so exhausted and I just remember
sitting by his bed and he said, he said, "Doctor K, have all the
patients in the private hospitals gotten out?" And I said, "Yeah,
you know what, they have." And he said, "Do you think, do you
think we're gonna get out today?" Now this is already going on

five days, an' I said, "You know what? I look out, the sun is setting, they've given us a lot of promises about coming, but I see the
sun is setting an' I think we're going to be here another night."
And I said, "I think we have to be prepared for that." And I said,
"I don't know, we might be here more than one night, I really
don't know." And he said, "Do you think that they are gonna
eventually come for us?" And I just said, "You know what? I just
don't really know."

And it made me feel just so crappy, you know, like—ashamed
a little bit? Like ashamed to be taking care of people and not to
be able to do for them what I wanted to do, which is get them the
hell out and get them to a, a safe place, you know?

I mean the patients at Charity, they're not dumb. The nurses
at Charity, they're not dumb. They *knew* we were gonna be the
last ones out. You know, they knew that the private hospitals were
gonna get private helicopters and, and you know it's, it's not, it
wasn't a, you know, it wasn't a shock to anybody. But the fact that
it wasn't a shock to people was so shocking to me.

You just see the, the desperation of, of being poor in this
country, and in some ways the distrust, I mean the, deep down—
that this is not the first time this has happened to people.

You know, I'm privileged and this is the first time I've ever
been totally fucking abandoned by my government, right? But
this wasn't the first time for my patients or the nurses or the other
people that worked at Charity Hospital.

I have a lot of history with the people on the floor, we all,
you know—I—a lot of them have known me since I'm a medical student and a hundred percent of our nurses on the floor
are African-American. What was really interesting to me early on
was that the African-American nurses and the other employees
at Charity *early on* said two things to me, which was, one: "They
open, opened the levees on us." 'Cause at first we were high
and dry. I could walk around outside the hospital. But when we
started to see the water rise, everybody said, we, and we all knew:
The levees broke. So they said, "They opened the levees on us,"
meaning they *flooded* the poor areas of Orleans Parish to spare the
other parts.

And then the other thing that people said to me *early on* was, "They're not gonna come get us. We're gonna be stuck here." And here I am coming from this privileged position in the world, "Well of course, what do you mean? They're not gonna come get us? What do you mean, of course, you know, FEMA—" They knew we were there, we were in constant contact with FEMA. "What do you mean they're not gonna come get us?"

And, our patients really did sense, and that part made me ashamed. *[And I thought]* it must feel like that your whole life: "You know what? We just have to do for ourselves because nobody is going to come get us." And that constant feeling of abandonment whereas for me it was all new. *Being abandoned.* You know, that was all new. But to so many people, it was just another thing. It was just another example of how they were abandoned.

And you know, people went about their business. Every, every nurse on our floor, they never stopped working, they worked for six days, in that heat, with no power, with flashlights. They never missed a vital sign. They never missed a urine output. They never missed a trick. And you know, there was this heavy sense of resignation.

[And] that feeling that I always tried to, you know, that kind of, that facade of, "Oh, you're here at Charity Hospital, but don't worry, you're gonna get the best possible care."

It was like that was gone, 'cause you know what? We are gonna give you the *best* possible care? But-we-can't-make-the-government-and-FEMA-come-and-get-us.

gence of new infectious diseases on a global basis that challenge us year in and year out, and those too can make a tremendous, a tremendous difference.

Drug companies on the news—largely offering the merits of, you know, sexual stimulants like Viagra—and paying little attention to vaccines or medications that have a benefit for the common illness.

Our priorities have obviously been skewed in the wrong direction.

The whole focus right now on health-care reform is largely an economic one? But underlying that is a huge set of cultural views and expectations.

The whole, uh, difficult challenge of, uh, if you will, rationing or regulating health care is going to have to be part of the public debate.

You know, when I hear the debate go on from members of our Congress, they'll say, "Well, I don't want you to tell me what my grandmother should get or what my mother should get." But the reality, ultimately, is each of us have to make some decisions about that. We do it in a way on an individual level? And then we slip into a kind of slippery slope with one parent or child or loved one saying, "Do this." When in fact, the "doing it" isn't going to result in any true long-term benefit.

What are our expectations of what constitutes reasonable care at both ends of the spectrum? At the beginning and toward the end is gonna have to be part of this public debate, because it tracks right back to the economics and what we're going to spend.

I think that discussion has to begin by a significant cultural frame shift, that is really quite encompassing.

You know, there, in addition to being a pediatrician I'm a, also an oncologist. There was a study done just a couple of years ago that asks if *oncologists*, how often did *they* introduce to their, um, patient, um, that they were at the end of known therapy.

Rare. Rarely done.

Rarely does the dialogue take place that, you know, we, we have expended a reasonable, a reasoned amount of treatment. And we need to move toward comfort and care.

And I think that's a cultural phenomenon that doesn't exist throughout the world. I mean you've traveled the world, Anna, and you know how people talk about death and dying in other societies. It's different than we do here.

The kind of discussion that I describe, that a doctor may need to have with her or his patient about death and dying, may be one that a *[medical]* student, or even a resident, never really has organized supervision around. Shocking. Isn't it? Shocking.

I think that there are probably at least two or more reasons that have contributed to why that doesn't happen as much as it should. One of which is, um, the lack of skill and sophistication. The other is, in some ways the, um, concern that if you begin to, um, move toward that discussion, that, uh, it, you're, give, taking away hope, you know, from a patient. And then a third, which I think is a hard one for me to say—but I think nonetheless that, uh, an honest reflection is, *(Brief pause)* that it takes a lot of time.

SUSAN YOUENS

Musicologist, University of Notre Dame

"Passing Bells"

With a glass of red wine. Texas accent, refined, meticulous enunciation. The adagio movement from Schubert's String Quintet in C Major *plays throughout.*

Well, if you mention the word mortality, the first place in *[Schubert's] Quintet* that I'm automatically going to think of is the adagio movement? The slow movement?

Now, Schubert lived in a city that has always been death-haunted. Vienna is the only city I know of that has a funeral museum? A museum for funeral coaches? And, uh, all, all of the funerary pomp—that was not only expended on the Hapsburg monarchs, but also on ordinary citizens who would compete with one another for magnificent burials of the dead. So Schubert had always been, I think, very attentive to death—because he was Viennese!

Now, sometime in late 1822, or early 1823, we don't know *when, how*, uh, we know nothing about the circumstances, but he contracted syphilis, which was the *AIDS* of the nineteenth century.

It was evidently a severe case. Schubert had known what his fate was going to be from the time he was twenty-five. Schubert knew the kind of fate that he would suffer if the syphilis reached, uh, the third stage? Which meant: either paralysis or insanity or both at once, uh, and it's, 'course there's no cure.

So, everything that he composes from late 1822 on is under the sign of death.

There's actually one very famous piece from September 1828, right after the *Quintet*: the andantino movement of his *A Major Piano Sonata*. It begins in a relative minor and very wistful, like the beginning of the adagio of the *String Quintet*. After which, there's what I can only call a *gigantic* temper tantrum. Music that is unlike *anything* else in the nineteenth century. It's like a *cataclysm* exploding, or a *Vesuvius*, uh, happening. And then, that cataclysm dies off, and you return, to a repetition of the beginning of the movement with the added feature of something called *das zügenglöcklein*, or "the passing bells."

Viennese parish churches would ring little bells, to alert their parishioners when someone in the parish was dying. So that everyone could stop and pray for whoever it was. They wouldn't know who it was! And Schubert, in these last years, rings-the-passing-bells over and over in his compositions.

The, the *rage* and the *blame* was certainly there. You can hear it in selected places in the music. But, it's always followed by putting the genie of anger back in the bottle.

I think facing, facing death in the way Schubert faced it in his last year requires an *adamantine* exercise of will—to insist on the creation of unmistakable beauty. And the creation of songs and works that are not about bitterness and cynicism and resentment.

(Pause, listening to a question.)

It *is* a miracle that we have it. Publishers were, of course, interested in making an Austrian shilling or two. So, what they wanted from

Schubert were the genres that would sell to the middle-class domestic market. So the publisher wasn't interested in the *Quintet*.

Schubert died on November 19th, 1828, just shy of his thirty-second birthday. And in that brief *[life]*time, he composed over a thousand works of music.

I don't think I would have liked Schubert. *(Pause)*

I would have *loved* him.

He—he's my Shakespeare.

EDUARDO BRUERA

Palliative Care, MD Anderson Cancer Center

"Existential Sadness"

A very handsome man, difficult-to-ascertain accent: Argentine? Sitting on a chair against a wall in a small office, feet on the low table in front of him, biting his nails, in Palliative Care at MD Anderson Cancer Center, Houston, Texas. Very pronounced enunciation.

The uncertainty, the fear, the sadness and so on. That can also be helped. So, it will always be one of the most difficult periods in our life when we come to the end of our lives. It is not plausible to turn dying into a picnic; it will never happen. We're not built to assume with a smile the end of our lives. Some of us will. But most of us will not.

Not, not everybody dies the same way. Some people have an easy death. Some people have a very difficult death. And that should not surprise us because . . . some of us have a very easy *life*. And some of us have a very difficult life.

Major stressors that happen to us before we face the ends of our lives include adolescence, divorces, losses of our own families, death of someone else who's near us, job losses, relocations. We have a trend to confront the end of our lives the way we have confronted those events. So, if we were depressed and took to the bed, we probably will do it again.

If we were angry, we'll probably be angry. If we denied the whole thing, we probably will deny the whole thing. If we blame someone else, we probably will do that, too. So it's . . . We're a little bit predictable in our repertoire of coping. And those of us who drink, will drink.

And those of us, who— So in the way we use the resources around us to cope with a devastating problem, we are a little bit more predictable than we would like to think.

There are stories about people selling all their belongings and getting a sailboat and going out to the Caribbean, but that's usually not what happens. We usually buy at the same supermarket, do the same routine, and then we die.

Yes. *(Slight pause)* Profound, existential sadness.

ANN RICHARDS

Former Governor, Texas
(1933–2006)

"Chi"

May 2006. In a fancy Houston, Texas, restaurant, evening. Eating Chilean sea bass, fresh rolls. (No alcohol.) Enjoying every morsel. Hearty appetite. Famous Texas accent.

But let's talk about something else, Anna. That I think is really important to say to you. I have two choices every day when I get up. I can feel *good* or I can feel *bad*. And a lot of what I feel is in my brain. So if I tell myself this is going to be a great day—and I know to live one day at a time now—then it's a better day! But if I tell myself—I am *not* going to buy into a sickness life. So when I get up in the morning, I say to myself, "This is going to be a good day." And even when it isn't, it's better. Because I am conscious that what I think has a whole lot to do with how I feel!

Want some bread?

Well, no. I was not the first woman governor of Texas. In the twenties, there was Pa Ferguson, and he was married to? *(Gesture to request audience response)*

Ma.

And Pa got impeached, and Ma—became governor. Now, she was the one when asked about bilingual education who said, "If the English language was good enough for Jesus Christ, it's good enough for everybody!"

In cancer, you have a team. I have a surgeon! I have an oncologist! I have a radiologist! There's so much collaboration and, you know, everyone knows everything about your case. There's not some glorified "God Doctor." Those "gods" are gone.

Thank heaven. Thank heaven.

Dr. Cox told me that I'm-the-first-person-in-the-world with esophageal cancer to get both proton therapy and chemotherapy at the same time.

I'm sure *[it's big money]*, but I don't know, you see? I've got so much insurance. If one doesn't cover it another one will, and another one will. It's lots of money, I'm sure. If—I mean, do you think most of the people in this country? They couldn't—they couldn't do what I do. They don't have that level of coverage. I'm just *so . . . lucky.*

The first thing I said was, "Thank God I can afford to do this."

My daughter Ellen has managed this entire thing so that I don't have to use up my *chi* doing that. That's what it is. That's your life force. That's your light. And you have to have every ounce of it to fight this physical thing that you have.

I go to this woman and she does what's called "energy work" with me? Isn't it wonderful? I just go to her for a tune-up. Sometimes I just go to her for a tune-up. So I was telling her one day that, just, I had a hell of a day. A guy had come in who just had to see me that day. Just a friend, he wanted some advice. And, you know, like it wouldn't wait. But there's also something about being indomitable, you know. So anyway he left, and another guy came up and he was there, and I had to go drive way the hell out to the north of town to do something. And by the time I got to her I was, I was really whipped. And she said, "Ann? You are using

up your chi! You're giving it away to all these other people. And
you have to save your chi. That's your mantra from now on."

So tonight's an exception, I am giving you, it's my natural
instinct to give you everything I've got. Well, I can't do that now
because I have to save what I can to beat this physical thing.
I mean, people call me up and I say, "I can't talk to you right now,
you're using up my chi."

And they've put me on a regimen. I can't shake hands. I can't
hug people. I made an exception of you tonight. I can't do all
the things that I did to be governor. It's just, I just can't do it.
I just say to people, "I'm so sorry I can't shake your hand. I'm on
chemotherapy." When people get in too close, I just step back.

I'd love for you to meet my oncologist. Her name is Dr.
Phan. She's Vietnamese. I said, "Dr. Phan, do you have children?"
She said, "No, I'm married to this hospital. You're—you're my
girrrl!" What could you ask better than that? The minute you see
her you know she's married to the hospital.

They assigned her to me. And I think they kind of handpick
doctors that they think will work best with patients. I don't think
I have any Republicans on my team.

LORRAINE COLEMAN

Retired Teacher, Anna Deavere Smith's Aunt

"Gloves"

Having difficulty walking. Serving the author and a guest salmon and salad on a table with table cloth and fine china. A cane nearby.

When people asked me what I wanted to be when I grow up I said, "I want to be like Esther!" *[Your Aunt Esther.]* And, you know, growing up. I was her baby!

She took me like her little girl. She would buy me *shoes.* I don't think I ever got my *pink socks.* When I was little all I used to talk about was I wanted *white shoes* and *pink socks!* In the thirties! And, you know, with eight children. Oh, I thought Esther was *hot stuff!*

(Phone rings. Ignoring it.)

I don't run to the phone anymore.

When Esther was in the nursing home, the last thing I heard her say— She was in the hospital and I don't think she . . . *[that]*

I could converse with her? But when I turned to leave she said, "You still got that big ass!" *(Pause)*

That was the last thing my sister said to me! But, of course, at that time I didn't know she was going to die. And I said to myself, "Just think, that's the-last-thing-my-sister-said-to-me!"

That's all I remember. I was walking out of the room and she said, "*You still got that big ass!*" That's the *last* thing I remember. That's the *last thing* I heard her say.

(Long pause.)

You know one thing that I miss? *(Brief pause)* When we were little, *[we]* didn't have gloves. But when we came home from school, *Mother* would be standing at the door. And she would put our hands underneath of her arms. You know, I miss that? *(Demonstrates by putting each of her own hands under opposite armpits)*

When I lost my sweetie, your Uncle Clarence— When Clarence died, Michael and I went down to Union *[Baptist]* Church. And this lady, Miss Effie—she lived to be a hundred and four— Miss Effie came over to me. And I said, "Oh, Effie, I wish my mother was here so I could put my hands under her arms." And she said, "Well, m'not your mother, but you can put your hands under my arms."

And there are times when I get down, that I wish that I had my mother to put my hands under her arms.

JOEL SIEGEL

ABC TV Movie Critic
(1943–2007)

"Three Thousand Years of
Being Kicked Around Europe"

May 2006 and June 2006. A hospital by the East River in New York City. Sitting in a wheelchair, hospital gown, talking on a cell phone, and eating a single green bean. Tennis shoes, jeans, New York team baseball cap, T-shirt lie in a clump on the floor.

And ABC News has really been *through* it with this stuff! My *God.* Everybody from David Westin, all the way on down, everybody knows, where I am—what I'm doing—what's going on. I *scheduled* this so I would be as *well* as possible on *Fridays.* So I'd be able to review the movies. They're hoping I don't get much sicker. I'm hoping I'll make, you know, Fridays through the summer, doing the movies. And-I'm-doing-my-best.

Cancer is a—cancer wins! Cancer is a *tough* disease! Cancer's right up there! I think cancer is stronger than Tyrannosaurus rex! *You* know. *(Laughs)*

The other, look *[at]* the other diseases that we beat! Tuberculosis, cancer's tougher. You know the blay, the play, bubonic *plague!*

Cancer's tougher! They're . . . each person's cancer is different. Like *snow*flakes.

The whole theory of chemo? Is they try to *kill* everything. It's like, you know, beating up your dog with a *stick [to kill the fleas]!* You know, I, it's, it's *terrible!*

Sorry, I'm eating a green bean.

(Listening.)

Never, in my *life,* thought of myself as tough. I was always the *last* kid chosen when we played football. Or baseball.

I'm pretty tough! Really *shocked* the shit out of me to discover that. I have no idea where it comes from. *[I]* like to say it comes from three thousand years of being kicked around Europe!

I wrote a joke. I think. You know, this is the ultimate. There is a category of joke: "old man don't have long to live" joke.

The most famous is George Burns, whose joke was, he was playing Las Vegas, and he's in his nineties. There's a knock on the door. It's this *gorgeous* chorus girl who says to him, "I've come to offer you super-sex." And George Burns says, "I'll take the soup."

Milton Berle's joke was, "I'm so old I'm afraid to order a three-minute egg."

My joke is, "I'm so near the end, I want the pill that *causes* premature ejaculation."

(Long pause.)

I act a lot. It's a *character* I play. Joel Siegel, the guy who's on television. The *real* Joel Siegel's a little bit sadder. And lonely.

(Pause.)

I *have* been depressed. But I'm not a depressed person.

And the way I feel. The way I describe the way I feel. The anxiety. It's like you're a little kid and you're going to school?

And there's someone in the bathroom waiting to beat you up?
And you have to go to the bathroom. That's the kind of anxiety
I feel. I feel that anxiety before I get tested.

(Pause.)

No. *[I don't pray.]* Wellllll, see—I'm *Jewish*. An' it's different. *Book*
learning. We learn that we don't ask God for things 'cause he's
not gonna give 'em to ya.

Prayer to me is *hoping* a lot. I-do-not-believe-in a God who
would in *any* way, interact, between me and my disease. I'm *very*
Jewish.

(Pause.)

I'm not very spiritual. In fact, I'm not spiritual at all.

(Pause. "Let Me Down Easy"? Pause.)

I like those words. I like 'em a lot.

I love the imagery. I see a hand, putting me into the ground,
and very gently moving away.

And I like that.

PETER GOMES

Reverend, Memorial Church, Harvard University
(1942–2011)

"Why Don't You Stick Around?"

African-American, with a "Harvard" accent that sounds British. A fine summer suit, bright striped shirt, tie, watch fob hanging from pocket, bright-colored silk handkerchief in the breast pocket, small round parson-like spectacles. Wearing a classic fine British vintage straw hat reminiscent of the early twentieth century. He tips his hat. Walks and sits in the course of this. Elegant hand gestures of someone who has spent a lot of time talking from a pulpit, and a lot of time communicating above the waist.

You know, we're sort of left there *[at the end]*. The medical people have departed. *They're* not going to stick around. They . . . In fact, I was a very young man and I had a parishioner dying in the hospital. And when it was clear, that the person wasn't going to recover, no more could be done, the doctor says, "We'll leave him to you now," to the clergy. And they went off to fight another battle. And part of me was really annoyed at that.

I thought, "Mm, cowards! Why don't you stick around?" And frankly, I was glad they were gone. There was a recognition almost that they had finished their function, but we hadn't finished ours. And that their job was to keep the person *here* with all the science and all the technology we produce. But when it was clear that *[the person was]* going to go away, we were the ones who were to see that they went. Conductors, as it were.

And, uh, the doctors resent the notion that they're leaving in defeat. Because death is a defeat for them. And so they have to go off and save somebody else! They don't want to be around at the moment . . . of expiration. One of the most important things you can do for somebody is-to-be-with-them-when-they-die. And medical people don't like that, so off they go!

My work is to make the movement from this life to the next one as *graceful and easy* for the dying as possible. Leaving is not done like *(Snapping)* that. It is, *(Makes an elegant and slow parabola with his hand)* whatever the opposite of arcing is. It's like that, and off you go. At least that's what they tell me anyway. It is not like pulling a switch. I don't know this from my own experiences obviously . . . One of the great fears that the dying have is that they're, they're leaving everything they know and they're going into some terrible void. Doesn't have to hurt. It's just nothingness. And one of the things that the minister or the priest can do, is to say, "You—are—known. Not just by us here." You will not be entering into some kind of clinical *nothingness*. I don't mean to say it like that. You, you keep the emphasis on the fact that, "You're surrounded by people who love you, and know you, and you're going to be with the One who created you, loves you and knows you." So, "Go in peace."

"Relax." *(Pause)* I don't ever say "relax," but I do try to construct this notion that we know what we're talking about and you'll soon find out. And it's a good thing.

And eventually, the person is gone. And then of course the hard work is dealing with all those who are left around the bedside. Because there is some inevitable sense: "We failed. We haven't done what we're supposed to do."

(Moves, as if to gravesite) At the grave, I read the Prayer Book Office: "I am the resurrection and the life." All that sort of stuff. "Ashes to ashes, dust to dust. This is it, folks!" I don't say it quite that way, but I, I always insist that the coffin be lowered away in the presence of everybody there. You know, the convention is the coffin is there and everybody leaves. And then the undertaker comes and does his thing. I insist that you see the box go-down-into-the-ground. You-need-to-know-that-this-is-a-form-of-finality. And my little homily is something like, "All that is mortal about brother or sister is in this box and it's going into the ground. And we cast ashes and dirt into here reminding us that this is where it all came from. And we will not meet again under these circumstances. So *cherish* the moment." I do say that. I say, "*Cherish the moment.*"

And since I have lots of Harvard funerals, on Harvard Hill— in Mount Auburn Cemetery—you stand on a hill and you look off. In the distance you see Cambridge. And I say, "There's something of a little village here in this cemetery. People who knew one another on Earth, who may or may not have loved one another. But here we all are, and here we all remain, here we end up."

So it means taking the measure of the days you have, taking-death-seriously. Because it *is* ultimate. And realizing that we have had something *precious*. And that we recall it regularly and faithfully when we visit the graves of those whom we love.

And *my* job is to try to urge them to come back! I, I say, "I don't want you to leave here full of terror and sadness and sorrow. I-want-you-to-know-that-this-is-the-place-where-you-come-back-to-recall-to-life-in-whatever-fashion-you-have, the person we sent off today."

I say, "Come here again, bring *flowers*. Remember your loved one."

TRUDY HOWELL

Director, Chance Orphanage, Johannesburg

"Don't Leave Them in the Dark"

August 2005. Johannesburg, South Africa. A very large, white South African woman on a couch in her office. South African accent.

Well, last year, we had about, I think, four or five babies and children that passed away. And this year, we've had one, uh, so far. What happens is, they phone me any time of the night and say, "This little kid is very, very sick." And I'll come and sit with the child until the child passes away. So I make sure that I'm here for every child. *(Slight pause)*

They don't know death. You know that, to me, that, that is how I see it. They don't know that they're dying. They, they just feel they're a very sick type-of-thing.

Um, the older children, the, the twelve year old and the fourteen year old that we've got here, we, we sit and talk to them the whole time about death. We had one child, Nomsa, um, that, that was here, um.

Charlayne *[Hunter-Gault]* from CNN, um, knew Nomsa very, very well. And um, I sat with *[Nomsa]* for days and hours and telling her about the virus, and telling her about death. And um, Nomsa knew that, that she was not going to make the weekend.

Nomsa came to see me the Friday afternoon, and she said to me that um, her mother was, her mother had visited her the night before. Now, I knew that her mother had passed away about six years prior to that. So I sat her down and I said to her, um, "What time did your mother visit you?" And she said, "No, it was late at night," and so I said, "Well, she'll, I'm so glad your mother visited you. If you see your mother tonight again, if she comes and visits again, you must tell her I said, 'Thank you very much, that I could look after you so long.'" And um, she said, "No, she will."

And the next morning, the Saturday morning, I came in here. And *[Nomsa]* was sitting on the, the, the stairs and she said, "No, Mother visited last night again." And her mother said that she must pack all her clothes, she's coming to fetch her. She's going home. And um, I promise you, it was, and I walked up, and I said to her, "Listen, did you tell your mother I said 'thank you very much'?" And she said, "Yes, and my mom says 'thank you very much.'"

Well, I got into her room, all her clothes were packed, was in plastic bags, and it was waiting for her.

That Sunday morning, about three o'clock, Nomsa passed away, and I made sure, um, I buried her next to her mommy. You know?

So, so her mother came and fetched her, you know so, and, and she was prepared for it. She knew she was going to die, she knew. And it's not a bad thing.

She was prepared, she was prepared to go. All her stuff was packed, all her teddy bears were packed, and we took everything. Her clothes, her teddy bears, everything. We put it with her, in her, in her coffin. You know, so, um. She, she, she went very happily. She was twelve years old. *(Pause)* I, I, I, I just tell them that there's different stages of, of life. You know, I say to them, "You get born, and sometimes when you're born, you're sick. And you've got this germ in your body that makes you very sick."

And we talk about the germ, and we talk of, we play, we play with the dolls. I sit on the carpet and I play with them, the dolls. And I say, this is this ugly germ, and it's going into the body and it's making this little child very sick. And sometimes this, this child has had enough, you know?

And then what happens is, then I start talking about death.

You, you know they're getting sicker. You know, this is the next stage, and they ask questions like, "What happens if I'm dead?" You know? And I say to them, "Nobody can answer that." And then they ask about God. And they ask about, "Do, can I, can I come and visit you again after I've died?" *(Upbeat, interested in the fact)* They always just want to say, "Can we come back to Chance after we're dead?" That type of thing. So I say to them, you know, um, "You will always be in my heart, even if you've passed away. You're always in my heart and you're always with me."

In any case, you know, so—don't leave them in the dark. Don't leave them in the dark.

MATTHIEU RICARD

Buddhist Monk, Author, French Translator for the Dalai Lama

"Teacup"

A French man, now living in Nepal. Picking up a Tibetan teacup filled with a little bit of water.

We prepare for death every second in a way. I mean in the Buddhist approach of a practitioner—we think of death all the time, but not at all in a morbid way. To give all its richness to every moment of life.

In the evening when someone is dead in Tibet, you put his cup upside down. His cup, like his teacup.

(Lifts the teacup and gently pours the water into an open hand. The water spills out on the floor.)

Finished.